BETTER SIGHT
WITHOUT GLASSES

A complete system of self-treatment for eye troubles
which enabled the author to discard the strongest glasses
possible to prescribe.

BETTER SIGHT WITHOUT GLASSES

by

HARRY BENJAMIN N.D.

THORSONS PUBLISHING GROUP

First published 1929
Second Edition 1938
Third Edition 1941
Fourth Edition (completely revised and reset) 1974
Fifth Edition 1984

British Library Cataloguing in Publication Data

Benjamin, Harry
Better sight without glasses.—5th ed.
1. Eye — Diseases and defects
I. Title
617.7'06   RE991

ISBN 0-7225-0930-8

*Published by Thorsons Publishers Limited,
Wellingborough, Northamptonshire, NN8 2RQ, England.*

Printed in Great Britain by
Richard Clay Limited, Bungay, Suffolk.

8   10   12   14   15   13   11   9

DEDICATION

It is with a feeling of deep appreciation that the author acknowledges the personal benefit received from putting into effect the principles underlying the Bates Method, as outlined in the book *Perfect Sight Without Glasses* by Dr W. H. Bates, of New York.

Note to reader

Before following the self-help advice given in this book readers are earnestly urged to give careful consideration to the nature of their particular health problem, and to consult a competent physician if in any doubt. This book should not be regarded as a substitute for professional medical treatment, and whilst every care is taken to ensure the accuracy of the content, the author and the publishers cannot accept legal responsibility for any problem arising out of the experimentation with the methods described.

CONTENTS

FOREWORD

In giving me the pleasure and privilege of writing a foreword to his book on natural methods of dealing with visual troubles, Mr Benjamin has also given me an opportunity to say how widespread is the need for such a system as he advocates.

I have for long been aware of the shortcomings of the Bates System, laudable and beneficial as it may be. Many of my patients have acknowledged failure to benefit by its use, until, under my care, they were enabled to so cleanse the tissues of their bodies that they were eventually able to secure the best results.

Mr Benjamin states that many cases of eye trouble have been cleared up by means of the fasting cure only, and this I can bear out entirely. After a fairly long fast, many of those people who have been in the habit of wearing eye-glasses have either been able to dispense with them altogether, or have had to have them changed for less strong ones.

The complete system of treatment outlined so ably in this book by Mr Benjamin, will enable very many people to overcome most difficult and obstinate cases of eye trouble, provided patience and perseverance are devoted to the task.

That such a book as this is wanted, has been shown by the widespread interest which arose out of the publication of a series of articles by Mr Benjamin in *Health For All*, and I feel sure that in this, his first book, he will meet with a measure of success usually denied to budding aspirants to fame. In any case, he may be sure that his book will achieve a vast amount of good.

STANLEY LIEF

PUBLISHER'S PREFACE

The success of this book is borne out by the fact that it is now in its fifth edition after many reprints; and the continuing demand for it is an indication of the effectiveness of the methods it outlines.

It has regretfully become normal practice to deal with defective vision by immediately clamping a pair of glasses on the sufferer's face, and – judging by the number of bespectacled people – it seems that we have almost reached the stage in this age of television and artificial light where the wearing of glasses has become synonymous with growing up.

But, over half-a-century ago Dr W. H. Bates, a New York ophthalmologist, put forward his famous method of eye treatment, and it is by augmenting the Bates Method with sound Naturopathic principles that the author of this book set out to offer a more natural and acceptable way to better sight, thereby giving an opportunity for the many of us who are perhaps unnecessarily committed to glasses to cast off our 'crutches'.

AUTHOR'S PREFACE
TO FIRST EDITION

As nothing is so convincing as actual personal experience, I think it will be of interest to the readers of this book if the following short autobiographical sketch of my own life is prefaced to it.

It states briefly and without any attempt at flourish how I nearly entered the valley of the shadow of blindness and was rescued therefrom by the methods set out in detail in the succeeding chapters.

My own success in overcoming the dread disability with which I was faced, should infuse all sufferers from defective vision with the hope of gaining genuine benefit from these revolutionary methods of eyesight training.

I cannot say whether I was actually born short-sighted or not, but at all events on the very first day I went to school – at the age of four – it was discovered that my vision was defective, and my mother was advised to have my eyes examined.

Accordingly, I was taken to the Westminster Ophthalmic Hospital, and it was disclosed upon examination that I had extreme myopia; I was ordered spectacles of -10 dioptres, and so at the age of five I began to wear glasses.

I kept on paying periodical visits to the hospital to see how my eyes were 'progressing', and every two or three years I had to have my spectacles changed for a stronger pair; until at the age of fifteen I was wearing -14 dioptres.

I had carried on with my ordinary education all the time, managing to see well enough with the glasses to do my school work, and eventually I left school to enter the Civil Service.

When I was seventeen there came a crisis; I had been used to studying a great deal (I had visions of becoming something some day), but suddenly I developed a haemorrhage in my left eye. At the same time my general health was affected, and I had greatly enlarged cervical glands, some of which were removed, together with my tonsils.

At the hospital it was discovered that my sight had become very much worse, and I was kept away from work for six months to rest my eyes. The glasses I was given to wear now were –18 dioptres, –4 dioptres stronger than formerly.

I carried on with the –18 glasses all through the war period in various government capacities, but in 1918 I was advised to give up clerical work altogether, as there was a danger of my losing my sight. This advice, by the way, came from a Harley Street specialist.

In accordance with his suggestion I looked around for a suitable outdoor occupation, but could only find one that offered any possibilities, namely, commercial travelling.

It was the last thing in the world that I wanted to do, but 'needs must where the devil drives' – so I became a commercial traveller.

I made one or two false starts to begin with but, fortunately for me, I soon struck oil and found an employer who understood and sympathized with me, so that he allowed me to carry on with my studies in philosophy, psychology and political science (which interested me most), somewhat to the detriment of my travelling activities.

During this time I paid annual visits to the specialist, and he gradually made it clear to me, year by year, that my sight was getting worse and worse – in spite of my open-air occupation – until at the age of 26 he furnished the strongest glasses possible for me:

Right eye: –20 sph. –3 cyl. 170°
Left eye: –20.5 sph. –3 cyl. 170°

At the same time he told me quite definitely that he

could do nothing more for me, that I was to give up reading – my greatest joy – altogether, and that I was to be very careful lest the retina of either eye became detached through an unexpected strain.

Quite a cheerful interview, wasn't it? However, I carried on much the same as usual, travelling all over the country, staying at the best hotels, and making quite a success of my occupation (thanks to my employer's kindness to me), but the thought of having to spend the rest of my life bereft of books and with the danger of total blindness always before me, produced a background for my hopes and aspirations which was far from encouraging.

I still continued my annual visits to Harley Street, and was always 'comforted' by the specialist's report as to my condition, until at the age of 28 I felt that my eyes could not possibly last much longer. My sight was failing rapidly – it was difficult to read or write anything, despite the enormously powerful glasses I was wearing. I had pains in my head at the slightest attempt to look at anything closely, and altogether I realized that something drastic would have to be done – but what? The specialist couldn't help me, he had told me so!

In March, 1926, I decided to throw up my job – which was bringing me in quite a handsome income – and go and live in the country, and it was just at that time that the miracle happened.

I was given a book to read, or rather to have read to me (I wasn't able to read myself), by a friend, entitled *Perfect Sight Without Glasses*, by W. H. Bates, M.D., of New York. This friend's brother had practised the Bates Method and had improved his sight tremendously, so I was told. I took the book home, my brother read it to me, and I saw immediately that Dr Bates' view as to the cause of defective vision and its cure was right; I knew it instinctively.

I could see that the Harley Street specialist, and the host of ophthalmologists and oculists who provide the world with glasses, were wrong and that Dr Bates was right.

Glasses would never 'cure' defective vision – they made

the eyes worse – and as long as one continued to wear them there was no possibility of ever regaining normal vision. The thing to do was to discard your glasses immediately, and to give your eyes a chance to do what they had been wanting to do all the time – namely, see, which the wearing of glasses had effectually prevented them from doing.

I paid a visit to a practitioner of the Bates Method in the West End of London to find out the best way to apply Dr Bates' principles, threw up my job, left off my glasses – after 23 years – and set about re-educating my eyes to see.

Imagine how I felt when I first left them off! I could hardly see anything, but in a few days I began to improve, and in a short time I was able to get about quite all right without any trouble. Of course, I was not able to read yet (in fact it took me over a year to reach that stage), and it was only through coming in contact with another practitioner of the Bates Method, who lived in Wales, that this came about.

I had been living for several months at a vegetarian guest house in the Cotswolds – I had been a vegetarian for some time then – but my eyes, although they had improved when I first started the Bates treatment, refused to respond any further.

Upon meeting this young man I decided to go and stay with him for a few weeks in Cardiff and carry on under his directions.

He at once put me on a sensible Naturopathic diet – fruit, salads, etc., – and took me actively in hand. In a few days my eyes began to improve, and in a week I could actually read a few words. By the end of three weeks I was able to read – very slowly and painfully – my first book without glasses.

It is now two-and-a-half years since I left off my glasses, and I am able to read and write quite well. My distance vision is not so good, but I see sufficiently well to be able to get about all over the place with ease and comfort. My health and general appearance are infinitely better than they have ever been, and I am pleased to say that through the help and advice given to me by my friend, the Bates practitioner in Cardiff, I determined to take up the practice of Naturopathy.

To that end I studied hard to familiarize myself with the theory and practice of Naturopathy, and have completed a course of private study under one of the best known London naturopaths.

Since then I have started in practice as a practitioner of natural methods of eye treatment.

What a contrast to my position three years ago! What a triumph for Naturopathic methods of treatment!

HARRY BENJAMIN
London, 1929

INTRODUCTION

Defective vision is more prevalent today than at any time before; a state of affairs which has been brought about chiefly by the increasing dependence upon artificial lighting and the widespread habits of television watching. And, since the situation is likely to get worse rather than improve, it is reasonable to assume that the incidence of defective vision will continue to increase with progressively greater rapidity.

The answer to this problem has been the provision of spectacles, but this artificial remedy does not succeed in checking this ever-growing menace to the nation's health since such a solution is merely palliative. Indeed, no one expects to *cure* defective vision by the aid of spectacles – the most they can be said to do is to enable the sufferer to get about with as little discomfort as possible.

Many people will agree that these aids to vision are disfiguring and unbeautiful in themselves; there is always the danger of their breaking and causing injury to the wearer; they prevent many people from participating in athletics and social pastimes generally. Yet, in spite of all this, spectacles are regarded as a boon and a blessing to man, and, in fact, as one of the great achievements of civilization.

It is quite easy to understand the high esteem in which glasses are held, as without them millions of people would be unable to get about as they do, and more and more are resorting to their aid every day; but this is because the public has come to believe that defective vision is incurable, and that the only possible remedy is the wearing of spectacles.

If, however, it were brought home to these millions of sufferers from eye troubles (as I hope to do in this volume) that by wearing glasses they may be permanently preventing themselves from removing their eye defects, and, in fact, tending to make their disability worse, then the popular belief in the efficacy and necessity for these visual 'crutches' will begin to fade, and be replaced by a growing realization that what they had hitherto regarded as one of the wonders of science is a handicap rather than an aid to better vision.

The belief in the value and necessity of spectacles in all cases of defective vision is firmly rooted in the public mind. It is based upon the assumption that most defects of vision are due to permanent changes in the shape of the eye, and that, therefore, all that can be done is to alleviate the conditions by the prescription of suitable lenses.

However, thanks to the researches of Dr W. H. Bates, of New York, extending over a period of thirty years, there has come into existence a new school of thought regarding the cause and cure of defective vision, and the founders of this movement have concluded that defective vision is *not* generally due to *permanent* changes in the shape of the eye, but only to *functional* derangements that are capable of being overcome in many cases by simple, natural methods of treatment which forbid the wearing of glasses.

It will thus be seen that the treatment of defective vision is being carried out today by two rival schools – those who follow the old methods of reasoning and regard defective vision as in itself incurable, but capable of being alleviated; and those who realize that these defects are due to a number of causes, most of them capable of being overcome, and that far from defective vision being incurable, there is every hope of being able to help the sufferer really to improve his sight and often to regain *completely* normal vision, without having recourse to any but the most natural and simple methods.

To Dr Bates (a New York ophthalmologist, and one-time examiner of the eyes of children attending the New

York schools) belongs the honour of being the founder of this method of eye treatment (known as the 'Bates Method'), and by numerous experiments and demonstrations he has made it clear that many widely accepted views regarding the nature of defective vision are entirely fallacious. He has triumphantly vindicated his claim by restoring to normal vision thousands of sufferers who had been pronounced by the greatest eye specialists as incurable!

The Bates Method is now being practised in several countries with great success, but the work of Dr Bates has been completely ignored by his fellow oculists; in fact, he was persecuted in New York by the American medical profession for his unorthodox theories, and died, a medical outcast, a few years after this book was first published. Thus, there seems little likelihood of these epoch-making discoveries reaching the public through ordinary channels.

It is left to people like myself, therefore, who have derived great benefit from the system, to sing its praises, in the hope of being able to bring it before the notice of other sufferers from defective vision, and in this way to make it known to them that, thanks to the great work of Dr Bates and his collaborators, they now have the chance to discard their glasses for ever, and set to work at once to bring back to their eyes the faculty of normal vision which is their birthright.

1.
HOW THE EYE WORKS

To fully understand the difference between the methods of reasoning of the new and old schools, it is necessary to have some knowledge of the anatomy and physiology of the eye, as the main point of divergence between these rival schools of thought lies in their interpretation of the phenomenon of accommodation. (The movement of the eye from a near to a distant object, or vice versa, is spoken of as accommodation.) So that the following brief sketch of the structure and function of the eye is esential:

The eye or eyeball is almost spherical in shape and about one inch in diameter. It consists of three layers or coats:

1. The Sclerotic, or outer layer;
2. The Choroid, or middle layer; and
3. The Retina, or inner layer.

The Sclerotic Layer is white and opalescent, except in its central portion, which is transparent and is called the *cornea*. Through the cornea light is transmitted to the eye.

The Choroid Layer contains the blood-vessels which carry the blood to and from the eye. Just behind the cornea the *choroid* becomes visible, and is called the *iris*, with the *pupil* in its centre. Directly behind the iris is the *crystalline lens* which catches the light as it passes through the pupil and focuses it upon the *retina*. Around the crystalline lens the choroid forms into folds known as the *ciliary processes*, which contain within them the *ciliary muscle*. The ciliary muscle is connected with the crystalline lens by means of a small ligament, so that the action of the

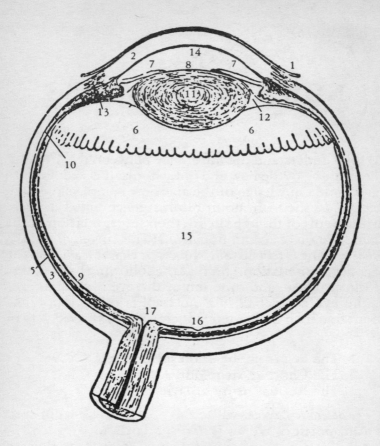

Fig. 1

VIEW OF THE HUMAN EYE, DIVIDED HORIZONTALLY, THROUGH THE MIDDLE

1. conjunctiva; 2. cornea; 3. sclerotic; 4. sheath of the optic nerve; 5. choroid; 6. ciliary processes; 7. iris; 8. pupil; 9. retina; 10. anterior limit of the retina; 11. crystalline lens; 12. suspensory ligament; 13. ciliary muscle; 14. aqueous chamber; 15. vitreous chamber; 16. yellow spot; 17. blind spot.

(From Furneaux & Smart's *Human Physiology*)

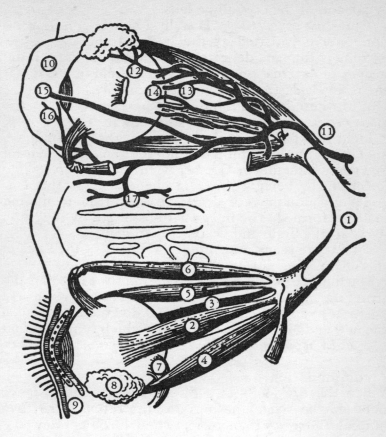

Fig. 2

VIEW OF THE EYEBALLS FROM ABOVE, SHOWING THE MUSCLES AND ARTERIES

1. optic nerve; 2. superior rectus muscle; 3. inferior rectus muscle; 4. external rectus muscle; 5. internal rectus muscle; 6. superior oblique muscle; 7. inferior oblique muscle; 8. lachrymal glands; 9. eyelid in section; 10. eyelid from inside; 11. infra-orbital artery; 12. branch to the tear gland; 13. branch to the retina; 14. branch to the iris; 15. branch to the upper eyelid; 16. branch to the eyebrow; 17. branch to the cavity of the nose.

ciliary muscle is able to control the contraction and expansion of the crystalline lens.

The *retina* or *inner layer* is really a continuation of the optic nerve (situated at the back of the eye); it is extremely thin and delicate, and upon it are thrown the images of external objects within the field of vision. (If the retina is destroyed, sight is impossible.)

With these facts in mind it will be easy to follow the *actual process of seeing*, which is as follows:

Light rays pass through the cornea, the external rays are cut off by the pupil, and only the remaining central rays really enter the eye. These pass through the crystalline lens, which, being convex in shape, causes them to converge upon the retina with the result that an inverted image is formed. The image is transmitted by the optic nerve to the brain and vision is the result.

(If there is any interference with any of the links in this chain, then normal vision is impossible.)

Having grasped these necessary details regarding the structure and function of the eye, the reader is now in a position to appreciate the essential divergence between the new and old schools of thought which centres round the act of accommodation.

Accommodation

When the eye looks at a distant object, the distance between the crystalline lens and the retina is *less* than normal, and *greater* than normal when the object viewed is close to the individual.

The manner in which this change in distance between the lens and retina is brought about is explained in medical text-books as being due to the expansion and contraction of the crystalline lens, owing to the action upon it of the ciliary muscle.

According to this view the eye as a whole *does not change its shape* – only the crystalline lens.

The experiments of Dr Bates, however, have shown that *the shape of the eye does change during accommodation*, owing to the action of the *external muscles of the eyeball*, to which belong the power to move the eye about in all directions (up, down, sideways, etc.). It was found that these muscles move *the back of the eye* towards the crystalline lens when a distant object is being looked at, by means of the contraction of certain sets of the muscles in question, *thus shortening its shape, and lengthening its shape* when a near object has to be observed, in a manner similar to that of an adjusting camera.

When one realizes that *myopia* (short sight) is a condition in which the eyeball is lengthened, and *hypermetropia* (long sight), and *presbyopia* (old sight) conditions in which the eyeball is contracted along its longitudinal axis (the line between the crystalline lens and the retina is the longitudinal axis) it becomes at once clear that, from the standpoint of Dr Bates, these conditions are only the result of imperfect accommodation, owing to the faulty action of the external muscles of the eye. In the case of myopia the eye is kept definitely in a position which renders the seeing of *distant objects* difficult, and in the cases of hypermetropia and presbyopia the eye is kept in a position which renders the seeing of *near objects* difficult.

In short, Dr Bates' work brought him to the conclusion that *many cases of defective vision are the result of strain upon the external muscles of the eyes*, which in time cause the eyeball to change its shape.

This is the fundamental principle of the Bates System, and it is claimed that by employing methods to relieve the strain or tension upon these muscles many conditions of defective vision can be overcome.

In his book entitled *Perfect Sight Without Glasses* Dr Bates gives a detailed account of his experiments to prove his theory, and the diametric opposition of his view to that of the old school, together with the message of hope and encouragement it brings to all sufferers from defective vision, is amply borne out and justified by the wonderful successes achieved every day, both in America and in this country, by the Bates Method.

2.
WHY SPECTACLES ARE HARMFUL

It is, therefore, to the external muscles of the eye that we have to turn for a major cause of defective vision. In the past, these muscles have been looked upon as being of value only in helping the eye to turn from side to side and up and down, etc. That they actually cause the eye continuously to change its shape during the process of vision has not been generally appreciated, so that all attempts to find the cause of myopia, hypermetropia, etc., have led to the conclusion that these defects (known to be due to changes in the shape of the eyeball) must be organic (permanent) in character as a result of subjecting the eyes to conditions harmful to them – such as bad light, artificial light, cinemas, television, excessive reading, etc.

From the new point of view, however, it has been demonstrated again and again that bad conditions of work, etc., *cannot produce defective vision*. All that these conditions can do is to *aggravate* an already existing *tendency* to defective vision due to a strained and contracted condition of the external muscles of the eye, so that what is generally regarded as the *cause* of eye trouble is merely a secondary factor.

Not knowing the seat of the trouble, therefore, and assuming that once the eye becomes myopic, hyper-metropic, or presbyopic (as the case may be) there exist no means whereby the eye can be brought back to its normal condition, the optical profession has concerned itself merely with the problem of how best to help the sufferer to overcome his disability in a manner most convenient to himself, and to this end spectacles were introduced.

Having furnished the patient with suitable glasses, the eye specialist considers that he has done everything that lies within his power to cope with the defective eye condition – and so he has; but a moment's reflection will show that by enabling the wearer to see more clearly than formerly by their aid, and so leading him to conclude that his defect is overcome, spectacles lull the sufferer from defective vision into a state of false satisfaction.

He quite naturally imagines that if he can *see* better, then his eyes *must* be better, and it is only after wearing spectacles for years, and having to change them more and more frequently for stronger ones, that the truth is borne in upon him that, instead of *improving* his eyes, the constant wearing of spectacles has in fact mde them *worse*, and will continue to do so.

What, then, is the value of spectacles? At best they offer a quick and easy means of dealing with a deranged visual condition – but to look upon them as permanent *aids* to vision is quite unwarranted.

To see this point quite clearly it is only necessary to realize that, once spectacles are worn, the whole natural process of seeing is thrown out of gear.

The eye, instead of being allowed to accommodate for near and distant objects, has the accommodation done for it in a fixed and unchangeable way by the spectacles, with the result that the strained condition of the muscles (which prevented accommodation in the first place) is intensified by the eyes being thus held in a *rigid position* by the action of the glasses.

This explains why the continual reliance upon spectacles *often tends to make the eyes worse* – the cause of the trouble is not only *not removed*, but is aggravated and intensified by the introduction of these so-called 'aids to vision'; at the same time no attempt is made to alter the artificial conditions which impose a strain upon already strained muscles, and so we find, therefore, that the practice of prescribing glasses for defective vision is *in itself* a major

cause of the continued increase of the very condition it
set out to overcome.

Natural Treatment

Once the sufferer from defective vision has become
aware of the part played by spectacles in making permanent
what often would otherwise be but a temporary derangement of the process of vision (if treated by natural means)
he will be only too eager to become acquainted with these
new methods of treatment; but he will probably feel that
it would be asking too much to expect him to discard his
glasses immediately, and have to go through that initial
period of inconvenience which must necessarily elapse
between the time that treatment is commenced and
sufficient improvement has been made to enable him to
go about for good without their aid.

It is *not*, however, absolutely essential to give up
completely wearing glasses once the treatment is undertaken (although the best and quickest results are obtained
when this is done), and many patients have been cured of
defects of vision who have worn glasses most of the time
they were under treatment. They found that they had to
wear weaker and weaker pairs as the treatment progressed,
until there came a time when they were no longer
necessary!

Spectacles may be worn during treatment, but only for
the purpose of work, household duties, etc., and should
be left off during leisure hours and when the exercises and
various details comprising the treatment are to be carried
out. Even if glasses are only left off for a *few hours* each day,
this will enable the eyes to begin to act naturally, and after
a couple of weeks of treatment the patient will be
agreeably surprised at the improvement in his vision –
which will be made abundantly clear to him by the fact
that the glasses he is wearing have now probably become
too strong for him – and older and weaker pairs will have
to be raked out of drawers and cupboards in which they
have lain almost forgotten for years.

It will be seen, therefore, that the taking up of these

new methods of treatment does not hinder the patient in his daily routine, but that they are intended to be carried out in his spare time, in his own home, and when most convenient. Once the basis of treatment is explained, and instructions given to meet the requirements of the different forms of defective vision, the sufferer can set to work *at once* to improve his sight, and the reward of his efforts will be in the gradual and continual progress he will notice in his condition.

Naturally, it will depend upon the degree of defective vision present, and the length of time it has been allowed to progress, as to how quickly the return towards normal vision will be effected, because the longer glasses have been worn, the more time it will take to break down the strain set up by them, both in the eyes themselves, and in the muscles and nerves connected with them.

In most cases, however, if the natural treatment is faithfully and regularly carried out, *improvement must follow* - a statement which is fully justified by the gratifying results obtained by Bates practitioners, both in this and other countries.

3.
CAUSES OF DEFECTIVE VISION

In the preceding chapters the inadequacy of the old method of treating defective vision has been dealt with, and the cause of such defects as myopia, hypermetropia, presbyopia etc., has been definitely attributed to a strained condition of the muscles surrounding the eyes.

It is now necessary to consider how it is possible for the muscles in question to *become* strained and contracted, and when this is done the *underlying causes of defective vision* will be made apparent.

Mental Strain

Dr Bates states quite definitely that he considers the cause of all defects of vision to be *mental strain* which sets up a corresponding physical strain upon the eyes and their muscles and nerves – thus leading to defective vision.

He considers that a highly nervous temperament, with a tendency to mental tenseness and rigidity of thought, is the cause of most cases of serious visual deficiency, and he looks upon the lesser defects as being mainly due to strain upon the mind (and consequently the brain and nervous system) set up by overwork, worry, fear, anxiety, etc., the degree of defective vision in all cases varying with the temperament and nervous condition of the individual. In pursuance of this theory, Dr Bates has concentrated his efforts upon methods of treatment which will remove the condition of mental strain, and the keynote of the 'Bates Method' is therefore *relaxation*.

If the mind of the patient can be relaxed, then his eyes

(together with the muscles and nerves connected with them) will become relaxed in turn, and similarly, if the eyes and their muscles and nerves can be relaxed, then the brain (and consequently the mind) will become relaxed in turn; and so we see that the Bates method of treatment aims at *mental and physical relaxation*, and it is only when this complimentary condition of mind and body has been achieved that perfect vision is possible.

The wonderful success of his system shows that Dr Bates' view is, in the main, correct, but there are many cases (especially those of long standing) where improvement has been slow, and in some instances absent altogether. In the present writer's opinion, the failures of the system are due in the main to a neglect of physical factors of the greatest importance.

To imagine that only mental strain can set up a strained condition of the muscles of the eye is evidence of lack of understanding of the working of the human organism, because it is obvious that if the cause of defective vision is a strained external musculature of the eyes, then any factor (not only mental, but physical) likely to set up strain in these muscles is a *potential cause of defective vision*.

It is in ignoring these other possible causes of strain and tension that the Bates Method shows its limitations, and cannot therefore be rightly considered a *complete* system of natural treatment for defective vision.

It is the purpose of the present book, however, to remedy this deficiency, and so to introduce a comprehensive and all-embracing method capable of dealing with many kinds of eye trouble in the best and most logical manner.

Food
In seeking to discover possible physical causes of strained and contracted eye muscles it must be borne in mind that the eye is part of the body, and as such must share in any condition affecting the body as a whole (to look upon the eye as something apart – as capable of functioning completely by itself – is fallacious).

It is to factors likely to prove harmful to the whole

organism, therefore, that we must turn our attention in our quest.

It has been known for some time that such diseases as diabetes and nephritis (kidney disease) have an effect upon the eyes, and it is generally admitted by medical men that some cases of *cataract* are diabetic in origin. Also, most laymen know that spots before the eyes are an accompaniment of liver disturbances and digestive derangements; but the remarkably intimate relationship that exists between the eyes and every part of the body is as yet scarcely realized, except by those with a knowledge of the science of Iridology.

It has been the work of the pioneers of iridiagnosis to show that every change (whether functional or organic) in any organ or part of the body is reflected in the eyes by a change of colour in the portion of the iris which is directly connected with that organ or part.

This wonderful affinity between the iris of the eye and the rest of the body is the result of a marvellous network of intercommunication between the nerves of the eye and the autonomic and cerebro-spinal nervous systems.

If the eyes can be affected (and they are) by changing conditions in distant parts of the body, how much more so will this be the case when the whole organism is involved? Many practitioners of natural therapy have discovered that inflammatory conditions of the eyes, such as conjunctivitis, iritis, and keratitis, are not to be looked upon as diseases simply affecting the eyes and nothing else (as is a common practice among the medical profession), but as symptoms of a *general toxaemic condition* of the body – due to excessive starch, sugar, and protein ingestion mainly. At the same time they have come to realize that cataract is only a sign of a more deep-seated (and therefore chronic) manifestation of the same condition of affairs.

The writer's own experience has shown him that wrong feeding has an effect not only upon the eyes themselves (as has just been illustrated), but upon the actual processes whereby vision is accomplished (something quite different), because the muscles and blood-vessels surrounding the eyes share in the clogging process set up all over the body by imperfect metabolism due to an unbalanced and too concentrated dietary.

Once the muscles and blood-vessels become clogged, proper drainage is impossible, and in time the muscles, instead of being soft and pliable, become hard and contracted. This eventually has the effect of preventing perfect accommodation, and later the shape of the eye is affected as a direct consequence. The ultimate result is *defective vision*.

Many cases of simple myopia, hypermetropia, and astigmatism are due to no other cause than the above, whilst presbyopia (old sight) is *almost entirely* due to it.

Up to now it has been assumed that when a person reaches middle age the eyes naturally change their shape (becoming slightly contracted), thus making the seeing of *near* objects difficult, and causing presbyopia.

This is regarded as an inconvenient, but necessary, price we have to pay for being in the world so long! And the difficulty is overcome by the wearing of convex spectacles.

Very few of the millions suffering from old sight (or their medical advisers) realize that the *wrong feeding habits* of 45 or 50 years of living may be responsible for this change in their visual powers; but this is undoubtedly the case, and normal sight can be restored to many sufferers from presbyopia simply by the introduction of a sensible dietary and the carrying out of a few simple eye exercises.

To emphasize the vital relationship between food and vision, it needs only to be stated that there are on record many authentic cases of defective vision being cured simply by means of *fasting*.

The increased elimination induced by the fast has the effect of unlocking the accumulated stores of waste products which have been clogging the muscles and blood-vessels surrounding the eyes, and as a result the muscles are relaxed and vision improved.

Blood and Nerve Supply

The two chief causes of defective vision have now been dealt with – namely, *mental strain* and *wrong feeding*, but there is another and third factor capable of affecting the sight of the individual – this is an improper blood and nerve supply.

Unless the eyes are fully supplied with blood and nerve force, the process of vision cannot be carried out properly; and so any factor capable of interfering with either the blood-vessels or the nerves of the eyes is a possible cause of defective vision.

Of course it is understood that both mental strain and wrong feeding interfere with the proper blood and nerve supply to the eyes, but there are some purely mechanical ways in which this may be brought about.

The chief seat of mechanical interference with the blood and nerve supply to the eyes lies in the muscles covering the upper portion of the spine (at the back of the neck).

If these muscles become contracted or infiltrated they have the effect of pulling the vertebrae attached to them slightly out of place (producing what is known as sub-luxations), and these in time impede the direct flow of nerve force from the sympathetic nervous system to the eyes; in addition, the vasomotor nerves which control the size of the small arteries are affected – and so the blood supply to the head is restricted.

It is necessary, therefore, in all cases of defective vision to make sure that the muscles at the back of the neck are perfectly relaxed and loose, and that no spinal defects are present. To this end, spinal manipulation (either osteo-pathic or chiropractic) is extremely valuable; indeed, many cases of defective vision have been cured simply by spinal treatment alone. (This shows the great effect these contracted neck muscles have upon the blood and nerve supply to the eyes.)

Another point to realize is that in most cases of defective vision (no matter what the causes may be) the strain upon the eyes and their muscles, blood-vessels and nerves (mostly due to the constant use of spectacles) is transmitted to the muscles at the back of the neck, and these in turn become contracted. It may therefore be stated, as a general proposition, that sufferers from defective vision have stiff and contracted neck muscles.

It is now obvious that a complete return to normal vision is impossible unless these contracted neck muscles are relaxed, so that the value of suitable neck treatment is made abundantly clear by this consideration.

4.
TREATMENT OF DEFECTIVE VISION

Having made clear the various factors entering into the causation of defective vision, we now come to that part of the subject which deals with the methods employed in the natural treatment of these conditions.

As there are three main causes of defective vision, so there are three definite and distinct lines of approach to all cases undergoing natural treatment; but as it is impossible to state definitely whether any particular case is due to any one cause (it is more than likely that two or, perhaps, all three factors are involved) the most successful system of treatment will be that which deals effectively with all three of them at one and the same time.

Up to the present no such comprehensive system of treatment has existed. The Bates Method has concerned itself solely with the first factor – namely, *mental strain* – and has ignored the other two; practitioners of natural therapy who have attempted any treatment of defective vision have looked upon diet and fasting as the best methods of procedure – generally to the neglect of the Bates Method; and osteopaths and chiropractors, when dealing with patients suffering from eye troubles, merely resort to spinal manipulation and nothing more.

Each of these three natural methods of treatment has wonderful cures to its credit (especially the Bates Method), but there have also been failures, and the reason for this is obvious – they have all accentuated one factor to the exclusion of another, with the result that only in those cases which are definitely due to the factor being treated has a complete cure been possible.

A Comprehensive System

By personal experience the writer of this book has come to realize the value of all these three methods of treatment, and by incorporating their most valuable features under one head in the present volume, a really comprehensive and all-embracing system of treatment has been produced, a system capable of dealing in a practical manner with *any* type of visual defect (to the knowledge of the writer, for the first time in the history of the subject).

The instructions for the various exercises and measures to be carried out by the sufferer from defective vision are all designed with the object of enabling them to be performed in his own home, and at a time most convenient to himself.

It is manifestly impossible to give particulars for a diet suitable for all cases, or to more than stress the value of spinal treatment to all those in a position to secure this form of therapy where deemed necessary; but a chapter is being devoted to the subject of diet in general to enable the reader to gauge for himself a sensible dietary; and to help meet the requirements of those who find a course of spinal treatment beyond them, a number of remedial exercises are being set out to help loosen up contracted neck muscles (something of considerable value and importance to *every* reader of this book, in view of what has been said in this connection in the previous chapter).

It is hoped, therefore, that all those desirous of dealing with their visual defects by the methods set forth in the following pages, will bear in mind the possible threefold nature of the cause of their condition, and so pay as much attention to their diet and the exercises for relaxing the neck, as to the various methods whereby the eyes with their muscles and nerves may be relaxed – in this way only can a return to normal vision be made possible.

The Eyes and Relaxation

Before normal vision is possible, the eyes and their surrounding muscles and nerves must be completely relaxed. There must be an entire absence of strain, as this tends to keep the eyes *rigid* and *fixed* and produces *staring* – *the first sign of defective vision*.

The normal eye is *always moving* – *it is never still*; continuous movement of the eye is absolutely essential for its healthy action, and this is only attained by complete relaxation of all its parts.

To bring about this relaxed condition in the eyes of those suffering from defective vision, Dr Bates has introduced two most important methods of procedure known as *palming* and *swinging*, respectively. These are described, together with various physical methods of obtaining the same result, in the next chapter.

5.
AIDS TO RELAXATION

When asleep we rest our bodies and generate a new store of nerve force for the next day's use, but, in the case of organs below the normal in condition, no opportunity is provided for them to catch up with the more fortunate members of our vital economy.

Palming

It is necessary in such cases to resort to accessory methods of producing rest in the affected organ, and in the case of eyes in which there is a visual deficiency, *complete rest for half an hour* to *one hour,* or *more, each day*, is essential to induce a fuller and more conscious relaxation of the eyes and their surrounding tissues, than that brought about through the agency of sleep. We frequently rest our eyes during the day (especially when they are tired) by closing them for a moment and palming is only an improvement on this natural and unconscious process.

To palm (see Figure 3), it is necessary to sit, in as comfortable a position as possible, in an armchair, or on a settee; get yourself as relaxed as possible – feel as loose and comfortable as you can – then close your eyes and cover them with your hands, crossing them slightly so that the left palm is over the left eye and the right palm is over the right eye, both slightly cupped, and leaving sufficient space for the nose to be free. Do not press on the eyes themselves at all.

Then with your eyes completely covered in this manner, allow your elbows to drop on to your knees, keeping the knees fairly close together. This is a very comfortable

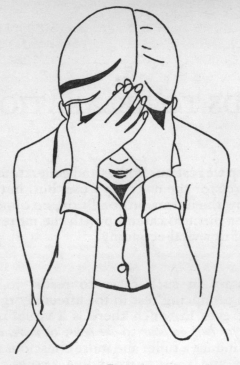

Fig. 3

position, and once it has been tried the reader will be able to assume it automatically, but if he prefers some other way of sitting whilst he is covering his eyes with his hands, he is at liberty to do so. *The great point is to have the eyes closed, and as relaxed as possible, and covered with the palms of the hands*.

In this way the eyes are rested much more effectively than by any other method, and the more black the colour that is seen when palming, the more relaxed is the state of the eyes.

The mind should be rested as well as the eyes, and to this end the patient should not dwell on subjects likely to affect him strongly, or think about the condition of his eyes, but he should either try to imagine the blackness that he sees growing blacker and blacker, or, if he prefers to, just let the mind wander as it likes over all sorts of pleasant and interesting subjects.

If this is done for ten, to twenty or thirty minutes twice or three times a day (according to the severity of the case) the improvement in vision soon to be noticed should be considerable, and this method of relaxation (or palming, as it is called) is one of the greatest assets to the natural treatment of defective vision.

Swinging

Palming directly rests and relaxes the eyes, but there is another method of inducing relaxation of the eyes and the surrounding tissues by its soothing and relaxing effect upon the whole nervous system. This has the effect of relaxing both mind and body simultaneously, and is immensely helpful in relieving eye strain.

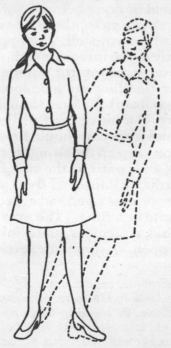

Fig. 4

This method is called *swinging* (see Figure 4) and is performed as follows:

Stand upright with your feet about 12 inches apart, hands loosely at the sides; then, keeping yourself as relaxed as possible, gently sway the *whole* body from side to side – imagine you are the pendulum of a clock, and move just as slowly. Raise each heel alternately from the ground, but not the rest of the foot. (Remember it is the *whole* body which has to sway gently to and fro, and not just the head and trunk; there should be no bending at the waist or hips.)

The gentle swaying, or swinging, has the effect of relaxing the whole nervous system, and should be practised two or three times a day for five to ten minutes each time, or whenever the eyes feel tired and aching.

Swinging should be done before a window,* and it will be noticed that as you sway, the window seems to move the opposite way from yourself. This opposite movement of objects directly in the foreground should be noted and encouraged. After swinging for a minute with the eyes open (always see that they are held loosely and relaxed, not rigidly and strained) the eyes should then be closed, and, *still swinging*, the movement of the window in the direction opposite from you should be *imagined* as clearly as possible, as you keep up the swinging movement. Then reopen the eyes, and continue the swinging with the eyes open for a further minute, and so on all the time alternating between eyes open and eyes closed, each for a period of a minute at a time. (The eyes must be kept as relaxed as possible, remember, and blink them every now and then when open, during the exercise.)

*Instead of a window the reader can substitute a picture or a clock or anything else suitable to vary the exercise. The window is here given because, on looking through it, whilst carrying out the swinging exercise, the movement of objects *outside* the window in the direction of the swing accentuates the *apparent* movement of the window in the opposite direction, and it is this *opposite* movement which is so necessary for the success of the exercise.

If performed correctly, this swinging exercise has a very beneficial effect indeed upon the eyes and nervous system, and is the best means (beside that of palming) of relieving eye strain.

(Of course, glasses should *never* be worn when either palming or swinging.)

Blinking

In addition to palming and swinging, there is a third method of producing relaxation of the eyes, and this is through the agency of *blinking*.

The normal eye blinks at regular intervals all the time it is open; it is done so rapidly, however, that we do not see it – but in those suffering from defective vision, the eyes become fixed and strained, and blinking, instead of being an unconscious and effortless process, is done consciously and with effort and spasmodically.

All sufferers from defective vision should therefore cultivate the habit of blinking frequently and regularly, thus preventing strain.

Learn to blink once or twice every ten seconds (but without effort), no matter what you may be doing at the time, and especially when reading.

This is a very simple but effective way of breaking up strain, and it will be found that a great deal more reading can be done in this manner than was formerly the case, and the eyes will be not nearly so tired.

Sunshine

The value of sunshine in all cases of defective vision is very great, and all sufferers are recommended to give their eyes as much of this as possible.

The best way is to *close* the eyes, face the sun, and gently move the head from side to side to ensure the rays falling on all parts of the eyes with equal strength. It should be done for about ten minutes three times a day, when possible.

This has the effect of drawing the blood to the eyes, and relaxing the muscles and nerves. (Glasses should *never* be worn when doing this.)

Cold Water

Cold water is very effective in toning-up the eyes and the surrounding tissues, and should be used as follows:

Whenever you wash yourself, before drying lean over the bowl, and, dipping your hands in the water (palms upwards and cupped), raise them full of water to within two inches of your *closed* eyes. Then splash the cold water on to your eyes smartly, but not violently. Repeat this about twenty times, then dry yourself and rub the closed eyes briskly for a minute or two with the towel.

This will make the eyes glow and it will freshen and tone them considerably. It is a very good plan to do it whenever the eyes feel tired, but, in any case, it should be performed at least three times a day. It is essential that the water should be cold, not tepid.

Special Note. As a result of recent experience with patients the author has found *Eyebright Extract* (Euphrasia Extract) to be of very great help indeed in toning-up and refreshing the eyes, as well as being of considerable value in cases of eye disease of various types. It can be secured through any homoeopathic chemist, and the dosage is three to five drops in an eye-bath of warm water. It can be used night and morning or just nightly, or whenever thought necessary. It is best to boil the water and then allow to cool off to warm before using.

6.
AIDS TO VISION

In the previous chapter the various methods of inducing relaxation of the eyes and overcoming staring and straining have been described, and we now come to those equally important measures whereby the actual vision of the individual is improved, and ultimate restoration of normal vision thus rendered possible. The first two of these aids to vision are *memory* and *imagination*.

The sense of sight is intimately bound up with the memory and imagination, and both of these factors play a larger part in the actual process of seeing than is generally realized.

Memory and Imagination
A familiar object is always more readily distinguished than an unfamiliar one, and this is simply because memory and imagination have come to our aid – the image of the object has been impressed on our mind through previous association, and the memory of these associations, plus the image, help us to pick it out more easily than an object seen for the first time.

Anyone can test the truth of this for himself – we can all distinguish friends among a group of people more easily than strangers.

In those suffering from defective vision, therefore, it is of great importance to cultivate the powers of memory and imagination, and this is done as follows:

Look at a small object (anything will do), observe its shape and size, run your eyes round the edge of it, and then, after getting as clear a mental picture as possible, close your eyes, and try to remember it as perfectly as you can. Open your eyes, look at the object again, and repeat as before. (This should be done for about five minutes daily, without wearing glasses, of course.)

A word in a book (or a letter in a word) is sometimes better for this purpose than an object. Imagine it as clearly and as black as you can, then close your eyes, keep the image before you, then open the eyes again. On looking at the word, or letter, it will appear blacker than before – a sign of improved vision. Repeat this several times, then go on to other letters or words.

The regular practice of this exercise is bound to lead to a noticeable improvement in vision in time. (The special Test Chart on page 94 is designed to facilitate the carrying out of the exercises enumerated above, and also those in connection with *central fixation* about to be described.)

Central Fixation

Central fixation really means *seeing best where you are looking*.

This may sound absurd, but those with defective vision *never* see best where they are looking.

Through the constant strain of glasses the central portion of the retina has become less capable of receiving images than the surrounding parts, because only the *central portion* is brought into use by these *artificial aids*. Consequently, when trying to see without glasses, those with defective vision will find that they can see better with the sides of their eyes than the centre. Only when the visual power of the central portion of the retina has been restored to normal (that is, when central fixation has been achieved) will normal sight be possible.

All the methods previously described help to bring this about, but there are other more definite ways of achieving it. The best is as follows:

Look at a line of print in a book, then concentrate upon one particular word in the centre of the line. Then close your eyes and imagine you see the line with the word in question more clearly defined and sharper in outline than the rest – let the rest be as blurred as they may be. Open your eyes, look at the word again, and repeat. Keep this up for about five minutes, trying to get the word in question clearer and clearer and the rest of the line more and more blurred as you go on.

You will soon find that the word *does actually become clearer* than the rest of the line – a sure sign of improved vision.

As vision improves, instead of a *word* in a *line*, select a *part* of a *word*. You can then keep on selecting smaller and smaller words and sections of words until you arrive at monosyllables. When you can imagine perfectly clearly one letter of a two-letter word, and the remaining letter quite blurred and indistinct, then *central fixation* is not far off.

Reading

The practice of *reading* is supposed to be responsible for much eye-strain, especially when carried out in a bad light; but, in point of fact, reading is one of the best ways of keeping the eyes active and healthy, and can never *cause* defective vision, no matter how much reading is done, providing the eyes are *relaxed* the whole time.

People with normal sight can read in any light without harm, but those whose vision is defective, and especially those who wear glasses, are subjecting their eyes to an additional strain every time they read.

In spite of this, however, one of the best ways to restore normal sight to those suffering from defective vision is to make them read (without glasses, of course) a fair amount every day.

If the reading is carried out properly, nothing but good can result, but if it is done in the usual manner, matters will be made worse than before.

The secret of successful reading is to *read without strain*, and this is accomplished as follows:

Palm for a few minutes, then take a book or newspaper and begin to read, *at the distance where you see the print best*.

(For those with *myopia*, this may be anything from twelve to six inches, and for those with *presbyopia* (old sight), two feet or more. In some cases of *extreme myopia*, it may be found necessary to read with *one eye at a time*, as the reading distance may be too short to allow both eyes being used simultaneously. In these cases it is better to cover one eye with an eye-shade whilst using the other, to avoid having to screw it up; the shade can then be transferred to the other eye when the first one is tired.)

Read a page or half-page, or a few lines, or a line, or even a few words, as the case may be, until you feel the eyes beginning to tire, then stop, close the eyes completely for a second or two, and begin again. Keep blinking regularly all the time you are reading, and in this way you will find yourself able to read *with ease* and *without strain*.

Reading, carried out in this manner, *improves vision*, and gives the eyes work that they want to do – it is their function to see – *but they must never be strained*.

It will, of course, depend upon the individual as to how long the reading may be carried on; but, in most cases, it will be found that in a very short time two or more hours can be managed without effort.

Those unfortunate ones who have to start with one eye at a time need not feel discouraged, for as they read with each eye, the one formerly used is allowed to have a rest. (In this way, with care, they can keep on for quite long periods.)

As time goes on they will find that their vision has improved and their focus increased – this will then allow both eyes being used together.

(Those with one eye weaker than the other should practise reading more with the weaker eye than with the stronger.)

No one with defective vision need be afraid to read whilst following out these instructions, and once it has become clear to the sufferer that he *can* read without his glasses, he will feel more than ever the desire to dispense with them altogether.

7.
EYE MUSCLE AND NECK EXERCISES

The following exercises are for the purpose of loosening up the strained and contracted muscles surrounding the eyes, which are rigid and stiff in all those suffering from defective vision. By making them supple and pliable the eye is allowed to move and accommodate more freely, and as a consequence the return to normal vision is greatly hastened.

The exercises should be performed whilst sitting comfortably in an armchair.

Exercise 1 (see Figure 5)

Keeping the head still and as relaxed as possible, gently allow the eyes to move up and down six times. The eyes should move slowly and regularly as far down as possible and then as far up as possible. Make no effort, just use the minimum of force.

As the muscles become more relaxed you will be able to look lower down and higher up as a consequence.

Repeat the six movements two or three times, with rests of a second or two between.

Exercise 2

Move the eyes from side to side as far as possible, without any force or effort, six times.

As in the former exercise, as the muscles begin to relax, you will be able to move them farther and more easily.

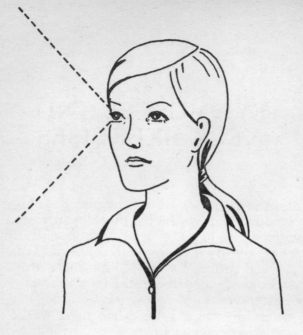

Fig. 5

Repeat two or three times, but remember never to use more than the *minimum of effort*, as the exercises are intended to overcome strain and *not* to increase it.

Rest for a second or two between the repetitions.

Exercise 3 (see Figure 6)

Hold up the index finger of the right hand about eight inches in front of the eyes, then look from the finger to any large object you like, **ten** or more feet away – the door will do, or a window.

Look from one to the other *ten times*, then *rest for a second*, and *repeat the ten glances two or three times*. Do this exercise fairly rapidly.

(This is the *best exercise* for improving accommodation, and it should be practised *as often as you like* and *where you like*.)

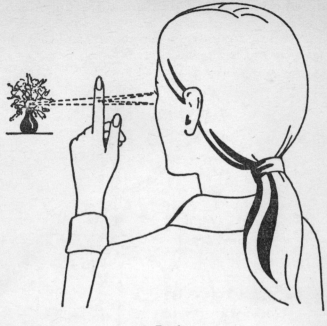

Fig.6

Exercise 4

Move the eyes gently and slowly around in a circle, then move them back in the *reverse direction. Do this four times in all.* Then *rest for a second*, and *repeat the four movements two or three times in all*, taking care to use the minimum of force or effort.

All the above-mentioned exercises should be carried out after *palming*, with a few seconds' palming between Exercises 1 and 2, 2 and 3, 3 and 4. (Glasses should *never* be worn at the time.)

Together, they should take about four or five minutes each day, and the improvement in vision that will follow will be ample repayment for the time spent on them.

Remedial Neck Exercises
The following exercises are designed for the purpose of loosening-up contracted neck muscles, and should be

performed even if a course of spinal treatment is being undertaken.

The best time to do them is on *rising*, and they should only *take four or five minutes altogether*.

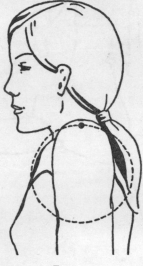

Fig.7

Exercise 1 (see Figure 7)

Stand as easily as you can, hands at the sides, then raise your shoulders as high as possible. Still keeping them raised, draw them as far back as you can, then lower them and return to the normal position, making a circular movement with the shoulders, fairly briskly.

Repeat this *twenty-five times*, making the movements one *continuous and circular rise and fall of the shoulders*.

Exercise 2

The same as Exercise 1, only in the reverse direction. Bring the shoulders back to begin with, then raise them as high as possible, bring them right forward, and then lower and return to the normal position.

Repeat twenty-five times in a continuous circular movement.

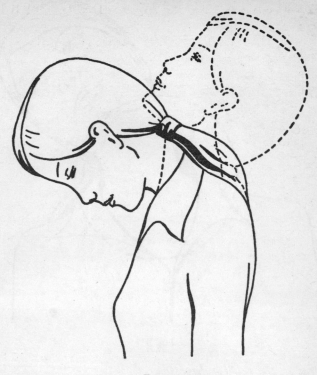

Fig. 8

Exercise 3 (see Figure 8)

Allow the chin to *drop as far forward as possible* on to the chest, *keeping the neck relaxed, not stiff*. Then raise the head and allow it to *fall as far backwards as possible* on to the shoulders and back.

Repeat twelve times.

Exercise 4 (see Figure 9)

Drop the chin forward on the chest as in the last exercise, then describe a complete circle with it – turning the head first over the right shoulder, then down over the back, next over the left shoulder, and return to the first position.

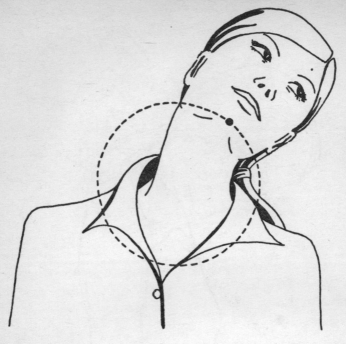

Fig. 9

Repeat in the reverse direction.
Describe twelve complete circles.
The neck must be kept relaxed all the time, and remember to reverse the direction each time, otherwise you may become giddy.

Exercise 5 (see Figure 10)

Turn the head as far to the left as possible, keeping the rest of the body quite still.

Return to the normal position and then turn the head as far as possible to the right.

Repeat ten times slowly.

These five exercises performed regularly every morning will soon ease the upper portion of the spine and neck, and in consequence a better blood and nerve supply to the head and eyes will follow.

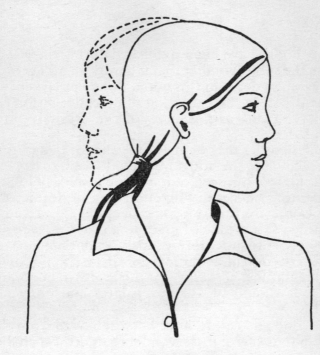

Fig. 10

8.
DIET

So many books have been published during the last few years on the subject of diet that it hardly seems necessary to refer to it in detail in this book, but diet plays such an important part in the causation of defective vision (and also in its cure) that a brief survey of its most vital points is essential.

We eat in order that we may live, and for that purpose food is taken into the body; but people seem to have lost sight of this sole purpose of food, and instead of looking upon eating as a necessary function to be performed with the same object as breathing and sleeping, it has come to be regarded as a means of gratifying our desires for the nice things of life (not merely satisfying our hunger), and the chief criterion of its value is not that it should contain the elements most necessary for the health of our bodies, but that it should please our palates and our senses generally.

Since food and eating have been removed from their proper sphere, it is of little wonder that, in most civilized countries today, there is a tendency to make articles of diet as artificial and as pleasing to the eye as possible.

This has led to the refining and demineralizing of sugar, bread and cereals (such as rice, barley, etc.), and to the preserving and potting of fruit, meat, fish, etc. There is a glut of such commodities as jams, cakes, chocolates, etc., to the neglect of natural foods, such as fresh fruits, salads, green vegetables and nuts, and where green vegetables *are* used as an article of diet they are invariably boiled, thus being denuded of their valuable salts and health-giving properties.

To those of us who have never thought about these matters, the artificial and refined foods we see all around us seem to be quite all right; and as everybody eats them and seems to thrive on them, why worry about them? Food is food, anyway!

On the surface this sounds all right, especially as some leading medical authorities tell us to *eat what we like*. But, during the last twenty or thirty years (thanks to the work of the pioneers of Naturopathy) it has become more and more evident that the artificial and concentrated dietary of the civilized portion of the globe is responsible for most of the serious diseases so vaguely attributed to 'germs' by the same medical authorities who tell us to eat what our fancy dictates.

Working from this basis, Naturopathy practitioners in America, Germany, and in this country have achieved remarkable success in overcoming such diseases as rheumatism, tuberculosis, diabetes, kidney disease, heart disease, etc., where the leading lights of professional medicine had given up the unhappy sufferers as incurable.

These cures have simply been effected by a sound understanding of the kinds of foods the body requires, and the best methods of combining them to ensure the greatest amount of benefit to the individual under treatment; together with simple, natural measures, such as cold water douches, cold packs, sun and air baths, etc.

The necessity for an understanding of this vitally important subject is, therefore, manifest to everyone, and no sufferer from defective vision can afford to ignore it. The main points to note are the following:

Natural, uncooked foods are the best to eat. These are: *Fresh fruits* (oranges, apples, grapes, peaches, plums, cherries, etc.). *Green vegetables* (lettuce, cabbage, spinach, endive, turnip tops, etc.). *Root vegetables* (potatoes, turnips, carrots, onions, beetroots, etc.). *Nuts* (Brazil, walnuts, etc.). *Dried fruits* (dates, raisins, figs). *Dairy products* (milk, cream, butter, cheese, eggs and honey).

The above-mentioned articles make the *best possible*

basis for a sensible, healthful diet, and all those who value their health, or wish to retain it, should see to it that these foods are well represented in their daily dietary.

There is no reason why people should not eat meat or fish, but they must be eaten very sparingly, and should be as fresh as possible. (No canned or preserved goods.)

Cereals are also necessary, but they likewise should only be eaten sparingly (once a day is quite enough) and for this purpose *genuine wholemeal bread* is the best and most suitable.

Jams, cakes, pastries, white sugar, white bread, confectionery, tea, coffee, etc., together with meat, fish, or eggs, two or three or four times each day, soon play havoc with our digestion and our bodies, and are, in truth, the basis of 'all the ills that flesh is heir to'.

The body cannot deal with them properly, and this leads to clogging of the tissues (skin, muscles, blood-vessels), irritation of nerves, and interferes with the functions of vital organs, such as the heart and liver.

As has been pointed out in a previous chapter, large numbers of cases of defective vision are either *caused* or *intensified* by years of subsistence on a diet too rich in starch, sugar and protein, and to ensure a complete return to normal vision, in addition to the various measures already described, a *revision of the dietary is absolutely essential*.

To help the reader, the following details should be borne in mind:

It is best to start the day on a *fruit meal*. Fresh fruit and/or dried fruit with *fresh cold milk* is the best breakfast possible. (No bread or cereal to be eaten with the fruit – just *fruit* and *milk*.)

Either at lunch or in the evening a *salad meal* should be taken, consisting of lettuce, celery, tomatoes, cucumber, watercress, grated raw carrot, etc., together with the wholemeal bread, butter, and cream cheese.

If any dressing is required for the salad, it should be *lemon juice* and *pure olive oil*. A second course may be stewed prunes and cream, or the like.

With two meals like this each day, the third meal may be anything within reason, such as meat, fish or egg with *steamed* vegetables. (*If potatoes are used they should always be baked in their jackets.*)

The second course may be dried fruit and nuts, baked apple and egg-and-milk custard, and so on.

Never use condiments or *drink with meals*. Cut down *tea* and *coffee* to a minimum. Make a point of having the *freshest food possible*. (No tinned or smoked fish, for example.) *Eat bread* only once a day.

If you *must* have tea in the afternoon, have it *very weak* and *without* sugar.

A diet composed on the above-mentioned lines will soon work wonders in a person's general health, and its effects upon the eyes, therefore, will be just as startling, especially if the other measures described in the previous chapters are carried out regularly and faithfully.

Special Note. The value of *Vitamin A* for improving visual powers needs stressing, especially for purposes of seeing in the *dark*. Maximum intake of this vitamin is most necessary as a daily measure in all cases of defective vision or eye diseases of any kind (most especially *night-blindness*). The best sources of supply of this vitamin are as follows:

In order of value: Cod liver oil, raw calf liver, raw ox liver; spinach (raw); rose hips, turnip tops (raw); dried apricots; cream cheese; parsley; mint; butter; vitaminized margarine; whale oil, egg yolk, prunes; tomatoes; Cheddar cheese; lettuce, carrots, watercress; cabbage; soya beans; green peas; wheatgerm; fresh milk; oranges; pasteurized milk; dates.

9.
HOW TO CARRY OUT THE TREATMENT

Having arrived thus far, the reader may be pardoned if he feels somewhat overwhelmed by the variety and number of methods comprising the natural treatment of defective vision, but if he is sufficiently determined to carry out the treatment, time can always be found for the work to be done.

Everything worth doing requires some trouble on the part of the doer, and the work of regaining normal vision is no exception to the rule.

All those intending to take up the treatment must be prepared, therefore, to make alterations in their daily routine to allow the carrying out of the various methods indicated.

This does *not* mean that they will be called upon to devote *all* their time to the treatment to the exclusion of everything else; but what *is* meant is that they must incorporate the various items into their daily lives – make the treatment *part of their lives*, and a most important part for the time being – in fact, until their goal is reached, and normal sight regained and firmly established.

The glasses formerly worn can then be relegated to the position of relics and curios, and exhibited to admiring friends as momentoes of a victory won over physical disability with the aid of *faith, patience* and *determination*.

The first requisite is *faith* in the efficacy of the treatment, and as far as that goes this book would never have been written if the writer had not come in contact with the methods of Dr Bates, and with their aid, rescued himself from the prospect of a life of total blindness and consequent physical incapability, with which he was threatened, despite all that orthodox medical science could do for him.

His ability to see now well enough to pen this volume is sufficient evidence of the value of the methods of treatment indicated in its pages, without referring to the hundreds of similar cases that can be quoted and are on record, and are a testimony to the wonders being worked every day by natural treatment both in America and in this country.

Faith in the treatment having been established, the other requisites are *patience* and *determination*, and with these as his helpers there is no obstacle insurmountable by the genuine trier.

It is beyond the scope of this book to give a detailed list of instructions to each individual, but for their help and guidance a typical case of each kind of common defect is about to be described and discussed in full, showing how the various measures to be employed are carried out, without interfering in any way with the daily work of the individual, in his or her *spare time* and *odd moments of leisure* throughout the day.

Everyone must regulate the treatment according to his or her environment and circumstances, but the examples given should prove an easy guide in the work of keeping up a daily régime. The results which follow will depend in each case upon the *seriousness of the defect, its duration, the temperament of the individual concerned* and the *thoroughness* with which the treatment is carried out.

In conclusion, it must always be borne in mind that once glasses have been dispensed with, the eyes must not be forced or strained by undue work placed upon them, and every care and attention must be given to them to build up their visual power, not only by the measures outlined in the present book, but by constant remembrance to avoid tension—both physical and mental—throughout the waking day. Otherwise, progress may be considerably hindered or even checked entirely in certain cases.

SPECIMEN CASES

Myopia

Miss A., aged 26, is a school mistress. She is suffering from *myopia* (short sight) and has worn glasses since the age of ten (during which time she has had to change her glasses frequently for stronger ones).

Like most myopic people, she is of a highly-strung and nervous disposition, always worrying about something, given to moods of introspection, and very fond of day-dreaming. These mental and emotional factors are the cause of her condition, which is further aggravated by a diet of the usual kind – too rich in starch, sugar and protein, and deficient in the natural foods like fruits and salads. In addition, the muscles at the back of the neck have become contracted as a result of the continual strain her nervous system is subjected to by the constant wearing of glasses – in this case for sixteen years.

In attempting to regain normal vision, therefore, the first thing she must do is to adopt a sensible form of diet along the lines laid down in this book, and having been told that the chief factor she will have to overcome in the course of her treatment is *herself*, she must begin to take things more calmly and easily, and keep herself as relaxed as possible.

She wears glasses only for her work, and has become used to getting about at home without them – this takes a day or two, but is soon accomplished.

Every morning on rising she performs the exercises for loosening-up the neck (which takes her only five minutes), and whenever she washes herself throughout the day, she splashes her eyes with cold water.

During the lunch-hour she finds time for twenty minutes' palming and ten minutes' swinging, and every evening after work she does a further half-hour's palming and ten minutes' swinging.

She cultivates her memory and imagination by looking at words and letters (without her glasses, of course) and imagining them as clearly as possible with her eyes closed.

She reads without her glasses for fifteen minutes a day to begin with, but this is soon lengthened to an hour, and later to two hours (with the help of blinking and resting her eyes every few lines).

As she reads, she holds the book farther and farther away to coax her eyes to increase their focus, and stops every now and then to encourage central fixation by imagining letters in a word clearer than the rest of the word. She then closes her eyes, keeps the image of the letter in her mind – the rest of the word being allowed to blur – and then opens them again and repeats several times (a procedure which helps her sight tremendously).

She goes through the exercises for the eye muscles in the train, on her way to work each morning, and when the opportunity occurs, allows the sun's rays to fall on her closed eyes for ten minutes at a time.

She finds her vision improving so rapidly that she takes to going out without her glasses, and to overcome her habit of day-dreaming (which sets up a strain upon the eyes) she looks at all the passing traffic, but without straining.

In this way her eyes are encouraged to see, and as she continues with the treatment she finds her glasses much too strong for her work, and so discards them altogether.

It is a bit difficult to manage her school work without them at first, but by using a much weaker pair of spectacles in cases of emergency, she is able to get along very well indeed.

She now looks forward with increasing confidence to the gradual restoration of her sight towards normal.

Hypermetropia

Alfred B., aged 14, has *hypermetropia* (long sight) as a result of complications set up when he was treated as a small boy for scarlet fever in the orthodox medical fashion, and has worn glasses for six years.

As soon as he begins treatment his parents put him upon a Naturopathic diet. He is encouraged to perform the neck exercises every night and morning, and splash his eyes frequently with cold water.

He still goes to school and wears his glasses only for his school work, being easily induced to leave them off for the rest of the day (he always detested wearing them), and on days when the sun is shining he allows the rays to fall on his closed eyes for ten minutes at a time.

He does fifteen minutes' palming morning and evening, and goes through the eye muscle exercises. Every evening he reads from a book as near as he can see the print without straining, stopping every few lines to rest his eyes, and blinking frequently and regularly all the time, but without effort.

In this way he finds he can read for quite long periods, and as he goes on, he manages, in time, to bring the book to normal reading distance from his eyes, which is about fifteen inches.

In a couple of months he has given up wearing glasses altogether, and can do his school work easily without them, but he still has to rest his eyes frequently to avoid getting them tired or strained.

His complete return to normal vision is now expected to be only a matter of weeks.

Astigmatism

Mr C. is a clerk, aged 30; he has astigmatism and has worn glasses for ten years. His trouble is due to the unequal pulling of the muscles surrounding the eyeball, and is the result of faulty dietetic habits in the first place, aggravated by constant work under artificial light – the clogged and contracted muscles being thus placed under a continuous strain. Neither of these causes of his condition was altered in any way by the glasses he wore – in fact, his eyes were getting worse, he found, and he had to change his glasses frequently.

In his case, the two chief essentials are a cleansing diet and the eye muscle exercises. He accordingly revises his diet along the lines laid down in the present book, and palms for ten minutes three times daily, following each bout of palming with the eye muscle exercises. He does the neck exercises night and morning, too, and splashes his eyes frequently with cold water. He leaves his glasses off altogether when at home.

In this way his vision soon improves, and in a short time he is able to work for several hours a day without his glasses, in spite of the artificial light.

He keeps up the treatment, and eventually has the satisfaction of knowing that his eyes are now normal again.

Presbyopia

Mr D., aged 54, has *presbyopia* (old sight). He is a salesman, and has never worn glasses, but finds his condition interferes with his work.

His trouble is directly caused by improper feeding habits, being used to a largely protein and starchy diet, and addicted to coffee drinking, and smoking.

He is at once placed on a sensible, natural diet, and encouraged to take plenty of exercise and look after his health generally.

He does fifteen minutes' palming twice a day and then the eye muscle exercises; after this he reads a newspaper as near as he can without straining, shaking the paper a little every now and then in order to make the print stand out more clearly, and blinking occasionally. He increases the time spent on reading as his eyes improve, which they do speedily as he keeps on with the treatment.

He performs the neck exercises night and morning as well, to help on his cure, and splashes his eyes with cold water several times daily, too. His progress is continuous, and in three weeks from the time he began treatment his sight is nearly back to normal. A further few weeks complete the cure.

Strabismus (squint)

Molly E., aged 7, has *internal strabismus* (squint) in her left eye, due to some of the muscles of the eye becoming partially atrophied as a result of nerve inhibition after she was treated for infantile paralysis in the usual suppressive medical manner.

She is instantly placed upon a fruit and salad diet, and given a course of spinal manipulation. This, together with the frequent shading of the right eye to allow only the weaker one to be used, soon works wonders.

She does twenty minutes' palming twice a day, performs the eye muscle exercises, and is encouraged to read as much as she can with the left eye (with frequent rests).

Special exercises are also given for the bad eye, with the other eye shaded. These consist of making her look at a pencil held before the eye and moved about, mainly towards the *right*, in order to make the eye turn *outwards*, as far as possible. This is done for a minute or two three times daily, the pencil being moved backwards and forwards in front of the eye all the time, with the patient following its movement as best she can, especially in the direction *away* from the squint.

As a result of all this, in two months her affected eye is found to be gradually coming back to normal and her general health is much better than it has been for years.

Cataract

Mrs F., aged 56, is suffering from cataract in both eyes.

Her trouble is only in the early stages, but she has been told that there is no cure for her condition, and all she can do is wait until the cataracts are 'ripe', when they can be removed by operation at the local hospital.

In the meantime, she hears about Naturopathic treatment and decides to give it a trial – not being at all anxious to undergo an operation, if it can be avoided.

It is explained to her that the cause of cataract is the silting up of the crystalline lens of the eye as a result of the lens becoming clogged with waste products – the residue of imperfect metabolism – and that it is a sign of a body full of poisons accumulated through the usual channels – wrong diet, and faulty elimination.

She is at once placed upon a very stringent natural diet, told to use an enema daily to clean out the bowels, and given some spinal treatment.

With regard to her eyes, she does half an hour's

palming twice a day, followed by the eye muscle exercises, and does the neck exercises night and morning. She splashes the eyes frequently with cold water, and sun-bathes them when possible for ten minutes at a time. She also does swinging for ten minutes daily, as she finds this helps her greatly.

Within a month she finds her sight beginning to improve and her general health as well, and is able to do more of the eye treatment than was at first possible.

She does some reading every day, also the *Memory and Imagination* and *Central Fixation* exercises, and is overjoyed to find her sight steadily coming back to her.

As the treatment is continued, her progress is so marked that she is able to see quite well with both eyes, and in addition her general health is better than it has been for years.

At the end of six months she realizes that natural treatment has not only restored her sight, but given her new life, and health as well, and she looks upon her escape from the operating table as nothing short of miraculous.

Special Note

The cases mentioned above are examples of the usual kinds of visual defects commonly met with in daily life, but it must not be imagined that only these are amenable to natural treatment. *Many other kinds of visual deficiency are capable of effective assistance from these methods, providing the case has not been allowed to progress too far,* and cures have been secured with *colour-blindness, night-blindness, nystagmus, amblyopia*, etc., as well as with the other types already mentioned.

In the following chapters, the cause and treatment of the most prevalent diseases of the eye are dealt with in detail, but before we turn to these conditions there are certain other eye affections which need some reference made about them. These are:

Detachment of the Retina. This is a condition which may arise through a blow or accident, or else as the result of extreme myopia and the constant wearing of very strong glasses. As regards treatment, palming for very long periods may be helpful to a certain extent, but most cases are unfortunately incapable of being helped to any marked degree by the methods outlined in the present book.

Floating Specks Before the Eyes. These are often due to physical derangements of function, such as liver and kidney disorders, and consequently need dietetic treatment to rectify matters; but other cases are due to the presence of particles of cell waste and other debris in the vitreous portion of the eye. They are of no pathological significance really, but often interfere with vision and cause annoyance. As regards treatment, a cleansing diet often proves beneficial here, but in most cases nothing can be done to get rid of the condition, and the sufferer is advised to forget about them as far as possible. It must, however, be recorded that the writer has been informed that *silica* taken in the form of *biochemic tissue salts* is often helpful in getting rid of floating specks caused by the presence of cell waste in the vitreous.

Styes. These are due to a run-down condition of the system, and therefore require constitutional treatment to get rid of them. Bathing with hot water and Epsom salts is beneficial, using a dessertspoonful of salts to half a pint of hot water. Be careful to keep the eyes closed whilst carrying out the bathing. (The use of *Eyebright Extract* may also be beneficial in these cases.)

Note on Biochemic Tissue Salts in the Treatment of Eye Diseases and Other Defects. The writer has subsequently investigated the value of biochemic tissue salts in the treatment of eye diseases and other eye defects, and feels it is his duty to inform his readers that much good has been secured by their use, in conjunction with the various measures set forth in the present book, in certain cases. These tissue salts are procurable at Health Food Stores, but require specialized supervision in their administration, and the writer therefore regrets that it is impossible to give a generalized scheme for their use by readers of the present book, whose condition might benefit from their utilization. One generalization can be permitted, however, and that is that *Kali. Phos.* is often useful for strengthening weak eye muscles and nerves, in conjunction with the system of eye treatment set forth in the present book.

Special Note on Night-Blindness. Research has revealed that *night-blindness* is mainly the result of an insufficiency of vitamin A in the diet. This vitamin is found most abundantly in cod- and other fish-liver oils, and in the other foods mentioned on page 61. Sufferers from *night-blindness* are therefore advised to take cod-liver oil daily, as a therapeutic measure, and also to include in their diet *each* day the other food items referred to, as far as this is practicable.

10.
CAUSE OF EYE DISEASES

Many people do not realize that diseases of the eyes and defective vision fall into two entirely different categories. Yet such is the case. Diseases of the eye occur as the outcome to pathological changes in the various eye structures, resulting from disturbance of function both in the eye itself and in other parts of the body. Defective vision is the result not of such pathological changes, but of a disability of the eye *as a whole* to accomodate itself to the instinctive physiological act of seeing. Shortsight, long sight, etc., are defects of vision; cataract, glaucoma, iritis, etc., are diseases of the eye.

Obviously, many diseases of the eye interfere with the processes of vision, and, indeed, sometimes succeed in preventing sight altogether; but that is only by the way, as it were. Primarily, they are not to be classed with those conditions through which the eye is prevented from focusing correctly for near and distant objects, and which give rise to what we call true defective vision.

A person with ordinarily normal health may develop defective vision, because the root cause of the defect is *mental strain*; but, for diseases of the eyes to develop, there must be something definitely wrong with the physical organism. We must never forget that the eyes are parts of the body, and as such they must share in any deficiency or disturbance of function affecting the whole organism; and, indeed, if we are going to put a finger on the root causes of eye diseases, that is the most important fact of all. *We do not have to look to the eyes themselves for the causes of eye diseases, but to the body as a whole of which the eyes form part!*

Orthodox treatment is based largely on the faulty assumption that because a disease affects the eyes, its cause can therefore be found in something which has only to do with the eyes, such as local irritation, prolonged eye-strain, etc. Such factors certainly play their part in producing diseases of the eyes, but they are only of secondary importance. Of infinitely more importance to the origin of eye diseases is the general bodily condition of the individual sufferer, and his past medical history.

It can be taken as axiomatic that no person who is in really good health can develop diseases of the eyes, such as conjunctivitis, cataract, etc. A lowered vitality and a poisoned bloodstream, due to wrong feeding and general wrong living, *are always* at the root of the trouble. Medical science tends to ignore these underlying factors; that is why its treatment for the conditions is so unsatisfactory. Constitutional treatment, and constitutional treatment *only*, can get rid of the diseases in a sane and satisfactory manner, leaving the sufferer in far better health than before, because of the thorough cleansing his system will have received as a result of the treatment.

Once the sufferer from an eye disease can be made to realize that he must look to the state of *his whole body* for the cause of his eye trouble, then he is already half-way towards a successful cure. It is only ignorance of that vital truth which prevents him from understanding his trouble and from being able to grapple with it successfully. The medical treatment for eye diseases is suppressive and unnatural, and it arises out of a fundamental inability to understand the primary causes concerned and in the development of the condition under treatment.

The most prominent of all eye diseases is cataract, and the medical treatment for that, by operation, is just as suppressive and harmful in character as any operation performed upon any other part of the body. It is merely the *effects* of the trouble which are dealt with, and not the causes. The constitutional condition of the sufferer, which is the key to the trouble in the first place, is ignored entirely by such treatment; indeed, the constitutional factor is aggravated.

Nothing could show more clearly the truth of the Naturopathic contention that the body is a unit, and in disease must be treated as such, than the gratifying success achieved in the natural treatment for eye diseases; such treatment is directed almost exclusively towards the cleansing of the body as a whole, although, of course, a certain amount of local treatment to the eye itself is given as well.

With that introduction to the cause and treatment of eye diseases, let us now turn to the actual diseases themselves and deal with them each in turn. (Only the more prevalent will be dealt with here.) The first, in alphabetical order, is *cataract*.

Cataract

Just behind the iris, or coloured portion of the eye, is situated the lens, through which the light travels into the interior of the eye. In cataract, that lens becomes opaque, and so the entrance of light into the eye is more and more seriously interfered with as the condition develops. When no light rays can enter the eye, through the opacity of the lens having developed to that extent, blindness ensues. The removal of the lens (or the major portion of it) by means of surgical operation is taken to be the only way of getting over the trouble; because, when suitable glasses are provided after the operation, the sufferer from cataract can see fairly well to get about and carry on his ordinary avocation, whatever it might be.

Once we assume that, if a cataract is forming in the eye of an individual, nothing can be done to prevent its future development, then perhaps the medical attitude towards the condition could be justified. Medical science waits until the cataract is 'ripe' (this may take a few years to bring about), and then the cataract is removed, and that is the end of the matter. The fact that the unfortunate sufferer has had to go about during the intervening years with his sight growing dimmer and dimmer, and with the prospect of a fairly serious operation always before him as something inevitable, is considered as something which cannot be helped in any way, things being as they are. But things need not be as they are, if only the treatment were concerned with the removal of the *causes* of disease, rather than merely its effects. For one thing, we know that people suffering from diabetes or Bright's disease sometimes develop cataract; surely that fact itself should throw some light on to the genesis of the condition as a whole? Cannot it be seen, merely from that, that constitutional factors are *always* concerned in the formation and development of cataract, whether Bright's disease or diabetes is present or not? The root cause of cataract is a toxic condition of the system due to continued wrong feeding and general wrong living; and constipation of long standing is almost always a predisposing factor in the case, just as it is with other highly toxic conditions, such as rheumatism. The blood-stream becomes full of toxic matter, which is carried through the body to find lodgment in any spot available to it. If, through strain, too prolonged use of the eyes, local irritation, etc., the lens happens to become defective in tone, the toxins will begin to exert their fateful influence there. As time goes on, the condition becomes more serious, and then cataract commences to develop. That, in brief, is the real genesis of cataract. It is a silting-up of the lens of the eye, over a period of years, as the gradual outcome, generally, of a highly toxic condition of the system. That practically all cataract sufferers are getting on in years, and have usually to their credit a past history of chronic disease, plus suppressive medical treatment by knife or drug, or both, are facts that only show how true is the contention we have made regarding the real cause of cataract. (Cataract in children is often the result of a diabetic condition of the mother during the pre-natal period.) The sufferer from cataract must not imagine, from what has been said, that his trouble can be readily cured by natural treatment, for cataract is a most stubborn condition to deal with. If cataract has been allowed to develop for many years, and has become deep-seated, nothing short of an operation will help matters. But, if the cataract is in the early stages, there is a possibility that the trouble can be got rid of by natural means; and even in fairly advanced cases it may often be prevented from becoming worse. (Surely the latter fact alone is worth something to the sufferer from cataract, haunted as he always is by the future prospect of a serious operation?) By a thorough course of natural treatment, to be described in the next chapter, the blood and tissues can be so cleansed that the cataract will disappear entirely in some cases of *early* cataract, whilst in many others it may be definitely prevented from becoming worse.

11.
TREATMENT OF CATARACT

We left off in the last chapter by saying that some cases of cataract, in the early stages, can be completely cured by natural methods of treatment, whilst others more advanced may be prevented by such treatment from going farther. Really serious and long-standing cases, we pointed out quite frankly, might have to face the possibility of an operation, even if natural measures were adopted, for in such cases it is more than likely that the cataract has too great a hold to be definitely dislodged.

It is very strange, but since writing that chapter, we received a copy of *The Homoeopathic World* from Mr J. Ellis Barker, the editor, in which he gave his own experiences in overcoming cataract by natural methods of treatment, after being assured by the leading oculists of the day that nothing but an operation (performed a few years hence) could save him from ultimate blindness! Perhaps a few quotations from Mr Barker's own words will be of interest:

. . . Some time ago I went to my optician in the West End to have my eyes tested. The usual reading tests were not satisfactory. Following them, the very experienced optician examined my eyes with the ophthalmoscope . . . After some hesitation, and looking at me in an embarrassed way, he said: 'I am afraid there is a peripheral opacity in both eyes.' 'Good God, is it cataract?' 'I cannot make up my mind whether it should be called cataract or not, but if I were you I would see a first-rate oculist.'

. . . I did not see a single oculist, but saw five or six who had been highly recommended to me by my friends. The first man told me quite bluntly that I had cataract on both eyes, that there was nothing for it but operation, and that it was awkward that the disease was equally strongly developed on both eyes, that, therefore, the sight of both would probably fail evenly. He informed me that there was no treatment for cataract except operation, that he could give me eye-drops or an ointment or such-like things if I wished for them, but that they were entirely useless. The other specialists told me that I had an opacity, or a cataractal opacity, or a cataract-like opacity, etc., but all agreed that nothing could be done except operation . . .

After being fitted out with new spectacles, and finding his eyes getting worse and worse, Mr Barker one day came into contact with a man who had proved for himself the benefits of natural methods of eye treatment in his own case, and he persuaded Mr Barker to see a practitioner of the newer methods of eye treatment. She examined his eyes and told him that she hoped to improve his sight immediately, if he would carry out the treatment. This is what Mr Barker says:

. . . I listened to her with the deepest scepticism. I said to myself that if it should indeed be possible to improve my eyes very greatly by exercises, etc., one of the five or six leading specialists I had consulted ought surely to be acquainted with the fact and ought to have told me what to do. However, a drowning man will clutch at a straw. I resolved to follow the lady's directions. That was about eight months ago . . .

. . . The change which has since then taken place in my eyesight is very striking. One might describe it as miraculous. Formerly I went out with four pairs of glasses – two pairs of reading glasses and two pairs of distance glasses – so that I should have a second pair of either should I lose one of them. I was absolutely dependent upon my glasses. And now – I have given up my distance glasses several months ago. Formerly I experienced eye-strain in going about without them. Now I experience very severe eye-strain if I try to use them. As regards reading, my experience has been more notable. In a good light I can read without glasses a book with medium-sized type or *The Times* for an hour or two without tiring. The other day, when returning from the Continent, I read during four or five consecutive hours in the train a book whilst my reading glasses remained in my pocket . . .

Some months after being under natural treatment, Mr Barker called upon one of the specialists who formerly examined his eyes for re-examination. This is what the dumb-founded medico said: '. . . I cannot understand it all. Your eyes have improved wonderfully since you came here, but they ought to have got worse, since you are considerably over sixty. You must not wear the glasses which I prescribed for you last time. They are far too strong for you . . .'

That, then, is the experience of Mr J. Ellis Barker, a man who is known far and wide as one who is always out for the truth where matters of health are concerned. Surely his experience with the newer methods of eye treatment will encourage many other sufferers from cataract and other eye defects to see what the methods can do in their cases, too?

Now, to continue with the self-treatment for cataract: the palming, swinging, neck exercises, eye muscle exercises, and other methods for relaxing and strengthening the eyes, as outlined in another part of this book, are the first essentials to the treatment. The patient must give as much of his time as he can to these during the day. Then comes the question of cleansing the system of the toxic matter responsible for the setting up of the cataract in the first place, as explained in the previous chapter. For this, a thorough course of eliminative treatment is required.

The best way to begin is to undertake a fast for from three to five or six days, on orange juice, or water, or both, according to the age and vitality of the patient. After this initial fast, a diet of a very restricted nature, along the following lines, should be carried out for a further ten to fourteen days:

Breakfast: Oranges or grapes.

Midday: Salad (raw) composed of any of the vegetables in season, attractively prepared. Dressing of olive-oil and lemon juice. *No vinegar. Dessert:* Raisins, prunes (soaked), figs, or dates.

Evening: Raw salad; *or*

One or two vegetables steamed in their own juices, such as spinach, cabbage, cauliflower, carrots, turnips. *(No potatoes).*

Finish the evening meal with a few nuts or some sweet fruit, such as apples, pears, grapes, etc.

No bread or any other article of diet may be added to the above list. Otherwise the whole value of the diet will be lost.

After ten to fourteen days on the above diet, the sufferer from cataract may the begin on a fuller diet, along these lines:

Breakfast: Any *fresh* fruits in season (except bananas).

Lunch: Large mixed salad with wholemeal bread, or crispbread, and butter. Or baked potato in jacket, with butter.

Evening: Two or three steamed vegetables (other than potatoes), with either egg or cheese or nuts. Grilled or steamed fish once a week; chicken once a week. No other meat. *Dessert:* Baked apple, stewed prunes, or some fresh fruit.

The short fast and period on the restricted diet should be resorted to again, say, two or three months after the treatment is begun; and yet again three months later, if necessary. The bowels should be cleansed nightly with the warm-water enema or gravity douche during the fast, and afterwards as necessary. *That is most important.*

A daily dry friction and rub-down is most helpful in toning-up the system and speeding-up elimination, and for the latter purpose, too, the hot Epsom salts bath, twice weekly, is a most helpful procedure (2 to 3 lb of salts in a bath of hot water). The *closed eyes* should also be bathed night and morning with hot water containing Epsom salts (a tablespoonful of salts to a large cupful of hot water). Give the eyes a good bathing each time, and be careful the eyes are *closed* all the time, not open.

Fresh air and gentle outdoor exercise, such as walking, are two essentials to the treatment which must not be neglected.

If the foregoing eliminative treatment is conscientiously carried out, in conjunction with the general eye treatment as outlined in detail earlier in this book, the sufferer from cataract should soon see visible signs of reward for his efforts; but, as already stressed, long-standing cases cannot possibly hope to reap as much benefit from the treatment as one of comparatively recent origin. However, in every case, patience and perseverance with the treatment will bring its due reward, both to the eyes and the system generally.

As the sufferer will now have realized, the diet factor is of the utmost importance in his case, and the more his daily dietary is made to consist of fruits and vegetables – nature's cleansing foods – the better will it be in every way. No white bread, sugar, cream, refined cereals (such as porridge, rice, tapioca, etc.), boiled potatoes, puddings and pies, or heavy, stodgy foods are to be eaten. No strong tea or coffee. No alcoholic beverages. No condiments, pickles, sauces, or other 'aids' to 'digestion'.

When one thinks of what alternative forms of treatment have to offer to the sufferer from cataract, surely it is well worth the latter's while giving the treatment here outlined a full trial to show what it can do.

Special Note: Elderly people and those in weak health should not attempt any strenuous fasting or strict dietetic treatment without advice from a competent authority. Those suffering from any heart troubles should also be very careful about attempting any rigorous dietetic treatment without proper advice. Sufferers from heart troubles should also avoid Epsom salts baths. After any bathing of the eyes with hot water and Epsom salts it is always best to sponge well with cold or cool water.

The cataract sufferer should bear in mind what has been said in the present edition about the value of

Eyebright Extract. Many sufferers from cataract have found its use night and morning most beneficial indeed. As regards the question of Epsom salts baths, should it prove difficult to obtain commercial Epsom salts, it is permissible to substitute 1 lb of washing soda for the quantity of Epsom salts mentioned. The refined Epsom salts may be used for bathing the *closed* eyes, of course, as before.

12.

CONJUNCTIVITIS

Continuing with the natural treatment for eye diseases, we now come to *conjunctivitis*, which is a very common form of eye trouble. It is caused by inflammation of the inner lining of the eyelids, or conjunctivae.

The main feature of the condition is redness and swelling of the lids, accompanied sometimes by a feeling as though there were something gritty in the eye. There is often a copious discharge of tears (or 'watering'), and sometimes, in more serious cases, there is pus formation.

The medical belief is that conjunctivitis is due to 'germ' infection or eye-strain. Certainly the evidence is clear that prolonged work under artificial light, or excessive use of the eyes in one way or another, predisposes towards the appearance of the trouble, but its root cause is systemic in origin, and is to be found in a general catarrhal condition of the system.

No one can develop conjunctivitis who is not in a condition of general toxaemia due to wrong feeding and general wrong living. The sufferer from conjunctivitis is one who is always having colds or other ailments indicative of a general catarrhal condition; and as catarrh is a pathological condition essentially connected with the mucous membrane – or inner lining – of the nose, throat, etc., it simply means that the general catarrhal condition of the mucous membranes concerned has spread to the mucous lining of the eyelids, too, and affected them also. That is the whole secret of conjunctivitis – that, and nothing more. One has, of course, always to keep in mind the possible accessory part played by eyestrain in weakening the tone of the eye-structures, and so bringing on the trouble.

Once we realize the true cause of conjunctivitis, the uselessness of so-called 'remedies' such as salves, ointments, etc., will be at once apparent to the intelligent reader. Treatment *must be constitutional*, if it is to be effective at all. The sufferer from conjunctivitis usually eats far too much starchy and sugary food in the shape of white bread, refined cereals, boiled potatoes, puddings, pies, pastry, sugar, jams, confectionery, etc. *Those* create the root cause of his general catarrhal condition (and conjunctivitis, too); especially when coupled, as they generally are, with the eating of excessive quantities of meat and other protein and fatty foods, the drinking of much strong tea and coffee, and the abuse of salt, condiments, sauces, and other seasonings.

We can also add to the above citation a rundown condition of the system, due to enervating habits and wrong-living generally, and a tendency to excessive use of the eyes under bad lighting conditions, or undue eye-strain to complete the picture.

It will be obvious from the above that only a thorough *internal* cleansing of the system, with the adoption of a future rational scheme of diet and general living, can help to get rid of conjunctivitis, once it has taken a hold upon the system. And the sufferer from the complaint who wishes to build up his whole system, as well as cure conjunctivitis, should take his own treatment in hand, and begin forthwith, as follows.

The best way to commence is to adopt an exclusively fresh-fruit diet for from seven to ten days. For that diet one has any *fresh* fruit in season, such as apples, pears, grapes, oranges, etc., *but no bananas*, and no other foodstuff whatever. For drinks during the all-fruit period, the patient may have only water, either hot or cold.

Those who have the trouble in a rather advanced form should have up to fourteen days on the all-fruit diet, to begin; or, better still, they should fast for four or five days, and follow the fast with fourteen days on the restricted diet outlined in the previous chapter on cataract.

The all-fruit diet, or fast and restricted diet, as the case may be, should be followed by a general scheme of diet along the following lines:

Breakfast: Fresh fruit, glass of cold or warm milk.

Lunch: Large salad, with wholemeal bread, and butter, or crispbread and butter. A few raisins or dates to follow.

Evening: Two or three steamed vegetables, with either egg or cheese or fish. Meat only very occasionally. (Potatoes, baked in their skins, twice weekly.) *Second course:* Prunes, or baked apples, or a little fresh fruit.

Note: No additions should be made to the above meals; but the midday and evening meals may be reversed, as desired.)

It will be necessary, in most cases, for the patient to have further short periods on the all-fruit diet at monthly intervals during the next few months, for two or three days each time. Those who have begun with the fast and restricted diet will need further fasts and periods on the said diet at two- or three-monthly intervals until the condition is quite cleared up.

It will be necessary, in all cases, to use the warm-water enema or gravity douche, nightly, to cleanse the bowels, during the first few days of the treatment, and afterwards, as necessary. (A clean colon has more to do with the clearing up of eye disorders than most people would imagine!)

All measures which tone up the system are useful as adjuncts to the above treatment, and a morning dry-friction rub and sponge-down, in conjunction with a daily exercise routine, including breathing exercises, will be most beneficial in all cases undergoing treatment. A hot Epsom salts bath, taken once or twice weekly, will also prove most beneficial. Fresh air and outdoor exercise are two essentials that must not be overlooked; as are also early hours, no excesses, etc. (With regard to the latter items, it is not our intention to preach a sermon, but the more closely the patient adheres to a scheme of clean, sensible living, the better will be the results that he will achieve from the treatment.)

As regards local treatment to the eyes themselves, the closed eyes should be bathed night and morning in hot water containing Epsom salts. (A tablespoonful of salts to a large cupful of hot water.) Be sure to keep the eyes well closed whilst bathing them. Exposure of the *closed eyes* to the rays of the sun, where at all possible, is also a most helpful measure where conjunctivitis is concerned. Of course, no salves, ointments, etc., are to be used in future. That goes without saying!

The eyes must be looked after carefully, and too much reading or too much close work under artificial light must be avoided. The exercises given in this book, for relaxing and strengthening the eyes, should be put into operation in conjunction with the general treatment here outlined. *Palming*, as outlined in Chapter Five, is particularly helpful in conjunctivitis. The patient should do, say, ten to fifteen minutes of palming several times a day, if he possibly can.

As already indicated, the diet factor is of extreme importance, and the more rigidly the dietetic instructions here given are carried out, the better will it be in every way as regards quickness of cure, future general health, etc. The items of diet previously mentioned as being the forerunners and direct causes of a catarrhal condition of the system, such as white bread, sugar, much meat, refined cereals, strong tea, etc., must be most carefully excluded from the future dietary, and fresh fruit and salads *must* form the bulk of the daily food. Otherwise, the catarrhal poisons at the back of conjunctivitis will never be completely eliminated from the system and so there will always be danger of the condition returning.

Special Note: See remarks in *Special Notes* at the end of *cataract*. Bathing with *Eyebright Extract* should be especially beneficial.

13.

GLAUCOMA

Glaucoma is a condition where there is tension in the eyeball, due to the presence of excess fluid. The eye becomes hard as a consequence of the presence of the excess fluid, and feels hard to the touch, instead of soft and resilient, as in the normal state. One of the first symptoms of the onset of the condition is the appearance of haloes or coloured rings round distant objects, when seen at night. The iris is usually pushed forward, and there is constant pain in the brow, the temple, the cheek, or other parts near the eye. There is also gradual impairment of vision as the condition develops, and ultimate blindness may ensue if proper steps to deal with the trouble are not inaugurated in the early stages.

Medical science offers severe eye-strain, or prolonged work under bad lighting conditions, as the main causes of glaucoma, although it is sometimes admitted that a general run-down condition of the patient has something to do with the onset of the trouble. But, in reality, the root cause lies much deeper than that. The basic cause of glaucoma is exactly the same as the cause of cataract; that is, a highly toxic condition of the system due to wrong feeding habits and general wrong living, plus suppressive medical treatment for previous disease, by knife or drug (or both) over a considerable period of time. Eye-strain is a supplementary factor only.

The medical treatment for glaucoma is operation, to relieve the internal pressure set up in the eye as a result of the presence of excess fluid. That, however, does nothing to get rid of the *cause* of the excess fluid. Consequently, even where an operation *has* been performed in glaucoma, it is no guarantee at all that the trouble will not return, or that it will not affect the other eye. Until the cause of the excess fluidity is understood and dealt with, a real cure is not at all possible, and operations must be recognized as being merely palliative at best.

The real treatment for glaucoma should be *constitutional* in character, not merely local and palliative.

As stated, glaucoma is a condition in which there is an excess of fluid in the eye, as a result of faulty eye drainage and congestion of the eye tissues. Now, when excess fluid appears in parts of the body other than the eye, it is recognized at once as being a sign of faulty systemic functioning; in other words, as an inability on the part of the organs of elimination to carry out their work properly. Excess fluid in the eye is no exception to that rule in the view of the naturopath, in the sense that the excessive fluid is taken to be a sign of bodily derangement of function due to a highly toxic general condition, plus imperfect local drainage. Of course, eye-strain and excessive use of the eyes in bad light, etc., are accepted as subsidiary causes; and a general run-down condition of the system due to overwork, excess of all kinds, etc., may contribute to the onset of the condition, which usually does not appear until the patient is well on in years.

The treatment for glaucoma, so far as Naturopathy is concerned, is no different from that for any other condition in which there is high toxicity; and the treatment for *cataract* (given in Chapter 11) can be followed out by the sufferer from glaucoma with some hope of good results being secured if taken in the early stages. Cases of advanced glaucoma may have progressed too far for the treatment to be really effective. Such cases may be beyond cure; but, even so, much can be done by the treatment to build up the general health-level of the patient, and for that reason alone the treatment is well worthwhile undertaking. Again, in advanced cases of glaucoma, as in cataract, even if a cure is not possible, the trouble can often be prevented from developing further by the carrying out of natural treatment.

If the patient is in a generally run-down and 'nervy' condition, a period of rest to begin the treatment is essential.

14.
IRITIS, KERATITIS, AND ULCERS

The iris, or coloured portion of the eye, is sometimes the seat of inflammation, which results in the condition known as iritis. Iritis is a most painful malady, and if this is left in orthodox hands may continue for many months, leaving behind it permanent damage to the sight of the sufferer. That is merely because the real underlying causes of the inflammation have not been understood, and suppressive measures, instead of eliminative measures, have been used as a basis of treatment.

Iritis is primarily due to a highly toxic condition of the system as a whole, and unless the *whole system* is treated, there is little hope of a successful termination to the complaint, so far as the complete restoration of vision and the general health of the eye are concerned. A person suffering from iritis is one who has generally a past medical history of disease of one kind or another extending back over many years, and, more often than not, long-standing constipation is one of the prime factors involved. To treat only the eyes and leave the general toxic condition untouched is a shortsighted policy when it comes to the practical treatment of disease.

For the effective treatment of iritis, fasting and strict dieting are the two measures most needed. It is only by a thorough internal cleansing of the system that the toxicity responsible for the condition can be cleared up, and normal health, both of eye and body, restored. The sufferer from iritis who wishes to follow out a scheme of natural treatment should therefore carry on as follows.

Begin with a fast of from three to five or even seven

days, according to the severity of the condition. During
the fast, only orange juice and water may be taken.
Nothing else. The fast can then be broken and the
following restricted diet begun:

Breakfast: Orange or grapes.

Lunch: Salad (raw), composed of any of the salad vegetables in season, attractively prepared. Dressing of olive
oil and lemon juice. *Dessert:* Raisins, prunes (soaked), figs,
or dates.

Evening: Raw salad; *or* one or two vegetables steamed in
their own juices, such as spinach, cabbage, cauliflower,
carrots, turnips, etc. (*no potatoes*). Finish the meal with a
few nuts or some sweet fruit, such as apples, pears,
grapes, etc.

*No bread or any other article of diet may be added to the above
list.*

The foregoing diet should be adhered to for from ten to
fourteen days, and then, if the condition has cleared up
sufficiently by that time, a fuller diet along the following
lines can be begun:

Breakfast: Any *fresh* fruit in season (except bananas).

Lunch: Large mixed salad, with wholemeal bread, or
crispbread, and butter. A few raisins, dates, or figs.

Evening: Two or three steamed vegetables, with either
egg or cheese. Grilled fish once a week. No meat at all.
(Potatoes, baked in their skins, twice weekly.) *Dessert:*
Baked apple, stewed prunes, or some fresh fruit.

If the trouble is not showing signs of definitely clearing
up after the fast and period of restricted dieting, a further
fast and period on the restricted diet may be undertaken
after spending a week on the full diet.

The use of the douche during the fasting period is most
essential to the success of the treatment, as long-standing
bowel trouble is one of the main predisposing causes of
iritis. The douche may be used twice daily for the first day
or two, and once daily thereafter, so long as the acute
symptoms of the trouble last. Afterwards it should only
be used as needed. A hot Epsom salts bath can be taken
three times weekly during the first part of the treatment

with excellent results; and the closed eyes should be bathed several times daily with hot water containing Epsom salts. (A tablespoonful of salts to a large cupful of hot water.) The eyes must be *closed* during the bathing. *Palming*, as described in Chapter 5, is often very helpful in cases of iritis, and should be done several times daily where found to give relief.

Future strict attention to diet, once the trouble has been overcome, is most essential; and care in the use of the eyes for close work, work in artificial light, etc., should be exercised for some considerable time to come.

Special Note: See also remarks made in *Special Notes* at end of treatment for *cataract*.

Keratitis

The causes which lead to the development of keratitis – or inflammation of the cornea of the eye – are very much the same as those for iritis just referred to. Keratitis, as iritis, is also indicative of a highly toxic general condition of the system, although eye-strain, injury to the eye, etc., are, of course, superficial predisposing factors to its occurrence.

As regards treatment, the sufferer from keratitis is referred to the treatment for iritis given in the present chapter. Such treatment should not only cure his eye trouble, but build up his whole general health, too.

Ulcers of the Cornea

The cornea is the sort of window in front of the eye which protects the pupil and iris. Not infrequently small ulcers appear upon the cornea, and give a considerable amount of trouble to the unfortunate sufferer. As with all other eye diseases, the cause of corneal ulcers is systemic in origin, and can be traced to wrong feeding in particular, and wrong living in general.

For an understanding of how a toxic condition of the system can affect the eyes, the sufferer from corneal ulcers is referred to the chapters on cataract and glaucoma; and as regards treatment, he can do no better than follow out the advice given for the cure of iritis and keratitis, if his case is fairly serious. If the case is a mild one, the treatment for conjunctivitis, given in Chapter 12, will be found to be all that is required to get the best results.

Strict attention to the future dietary is essential if further trouble of the same kind is to be prevented, and the whole general health-level should be built up by systematic exercise, hygienic living, etc. No drugs, lotions, etc., should be used as aids to treatment; the only local treatment to be employed being the frequent bathing of the *closed* eyes with hot water and Epsom salts, as advised in the treatment for all the other eye diseases, and the exposure of the *closed eyes* to the rays of the sun. *Palming*, as described in Chapter 5, is most helpful, and should be carried out several times daily, in fifteen- or twenty-minute periods. (The use of *Eyebright Extract* may be most helpful in conjunction with the general plan of treatment indicated).

Trachoma

Trachoma has not been included in this book because it is an eye disease which is not very common in this country. But all that has been said regarding conjunctivitis applies with more than double force to trachoma, for trachoma is a purulent form of conjunctivitis, with defective nutrition and unhygienic habits of living as its two main causative factors. As regards treatment, a protracted fast, or a series of shorter fasts, or fruit fasts, is the best way to proceed, followed by the adoption of a general fruit and salad diet as given for conjunctivitis, together with the carrying out of the general health measures therein advised.

TEST CHART

Fifty Feet

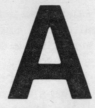

Thirty Feet

C G

Twenty Feet

F E P

Fifteen Feet

L Z O D

Ten Feet

C N G A B

Five Feet

H A Q O E

Three Feet

Z U K L T P A

Two Feet

B R O C G D N

INDEX